Losing Weight And Gaining Confidence

Deandra Barnhart

THE JOURNAL

How to lose weight and gain confidence without feeling like you have to be on a strict diet, taking away from the enjoyment of eating the foods you love, and losing weight without the pressure of over killing yourself with exercise. You can lose it with ease and actually enjoy it!

MY GOAL

To help woman and men gain confidence in themselves again to do exactly what they love and eat what they love without taking away from their everyday lives. Losing weight in a healthy way. Getting that confidence back in a matter of months.

The Plan

I have been searching for the easiest, quickest results in diet plans all across the world. I've tried fasting diets and all kinds of supplement pills to increase weight lost for instant results. Never found any that actually works or healthy ones that gave me good results. I also learned that losing weight too quickly wasn't healthy. I did my own research and finally found a plan that works for me. Something that gave me good results, kept me healthy and energetic. I still ate the foods that I love, didn't have to fast or use a strict diet plan, while losing pounds and inches in less than a year. Here's how...

Detoxing

The first trick to shedding pounds was herbs and herbal teas. Herbal teas/herbs are good for boosting metabolism. It cleanses you out and keeps you from bloating. It is also very safe and effective. Here are some good herbs and teas to use...

Herbs

Ginseng- Boost energy and speed metabolism (good for people with diabetes)

Cayenne Pepper- Shrink fat tissue

Mustard Seed- Burns calories

Cumin- Enhance brain function and good for stress relief

Cinnamon- Kills parasites

Nettle Leaf- Filled with antioxidants and vitamins

Sage- Reduce blood pressure and helps you to control eating

Oregano- Decrease bloating and constipation, also filled with antioxidants

Teas

Green tea, Herbal tea, Jasmine tea, Ginseng tea, Peppermint tea
[Ways to use them]
I sprinkle herbs in my food to boost the results along with the herbal teas I drink. I drink the tea 1-2 times a day. I made my own cocktail with a mixture of the herbs listed, in at least 8 oz of boiled water. Hot water is an inexpensive and effective way to lose weight. It is also good for your skin

Meal Plans

Don't be discouraged about "diet" plans. You do not have to cut out meats and all of your treats to lose weight; however you do have to regulate them. The first thing to do is cut back on red meats. Eat more white meats for the month and do red meats twice a month. For example: I like to do different things with chicken. For instance: Chicken Alfredo, Chicken Parmesan, Lemon Pepper Chicken, BBQ Chicken, Curry Chicken, Cajun chicken. For fish I would do Salmon, Trout, Tilapia, (baked or stuffed). Try to stay away from a lot of fried foods, which is bad for clogging arteries. Do spaghetti and steak for the month for example of red meat recipes, but no more than twice a month. When fixing your plate your starch should be the size of a toddler's fist while adding more greens on your plate. Always eat your meals with greens for weight lost. Drink plenty of water or coconut water to stay hydrated.

Vitamins & Minerals

Multivitamins are a must for weight lost. Your body needs it's nutrients for all the waste and toxins you put out. Teas can strip a lot from your body, such as iron. You can keep the necessary minerals in your body by what you eat. Here are some good fruits to snack on and enjoy, while getting the nutrients you need to stay healthy...

Apples- Contains: 195 mg of potassium
11mg of calcium
9 mg of magnesium
.22 mg of iron
.07 mg of zinc
.47 grams of protein

Avocado- Contains: 975 mg of potassium
58 mg of magnesium
24 mg of calcium
1.11 mg of zinc
4.02 grams of protein

Banana- Contains: 422 mg of

potassium
32 mg of magnesium
6mg of calcium
.31 mg of iron
.18 mg of zinc
1.29 grams of protein

Grapes- Contains: 288 mg of
potassium
11 mg of magnesium
15 mg of calcium
.54 mg of iron
.11 mg of zinc

Mango- Contains: 323 mg of
potassium
19 mg of magnesium
21 mg of calcium

.27 mg of iron
.08 mg of zinc

All of these fruits are high in vitamins A, B, C, D, E and K. Very helpful toward losing weight and boosting your metabolism as well.

Exercise

With all of the proper things I needed for my weight lost, I had enough energy to burn calories during the days of dieting. It took me 8 months to lose 40 lbs, without over killing myself with exercise. My advice would be, if you don't want to workout in a gym, use B12 vitamins to do your own at home workout. My favorite thing to do was walking. I did a 20 minute walk each day. Walking burns calories. I also did squats every 2 days (30 times) in the bathroom during my alone time. Squats help to keep toned around your butt and thighs. While walking I also contract my stomach muscles by sucking my stomach all the way in and exhaling repeatedly. That's a good exercise for those who hate doing sit-ups. For quicker results I would advise you to join a gym. You can run the treadmill, or work on any target areas you want better results in.

Maintenance

After I reached my goal, it became a habit to stick to my diet plan. I never eat too much red meats and I actually love eating fruits and veggies. Whenever I feel like I'm bloated I would make my hot water cocktail of herbs and grab an avocado to snack on. Avocados get rid of bloating. I kept sticking to my core target exercise of sucking my stomach in while walking, to keep my stomach down. Keep herbs on hand for food and cocktail drinks just in case you want quick results or you run out of tea. Drink the herbal teas, green teas. You can drink them hot or cold. If you decide to drink them cold, make sure it is freshly brewed. Drinking the tea cold does not make it ineffective, but to have better results add peppermint leaf in it. Use ginseng to boost energy during down time or when you feel sluggish. Laziness can pack on pounds. If you work at a desk or a slow paced environment, you can do the target core exercise while you're sitting or standing as well. If you are a busy worker, grab some oatmeal in the morning with lots of fruit in it or a granola bar with fruit a snack. Breakfast is the most important meal of the day. Oatmeal contains fiber which helps your digestive system and controls your metabolism as well. Snack on fruits and veggies throughout the day to get the vitamins and minerals you need.

Mission Accomplished

I hope this was informative to your dieting needs. I will be appreciative of any reviews, questions or concerns that you have on your journey of weight lost. Please feel free to follow me on Instagram @deandra.b my email is deandrabarnhart@gmail.com you can check my books out on amazon.com search by author Deandra Barnhart. Thank you for sharing this journey with me and God

Bless...